Essential Oils for Cough and Cold

Essential Oil Recipes for
Cough and Cold
for Diffusers, Roller Bottles,
Inhalers & more.

Rica V. Gadi

Printed in the United States of America

First Printing, 2018

ISBN: 9781792848858

http://eorecipes.net

This book is dedicated to all the strong people who are taking responsibility of your own well being and doing something to be better.

All my heartfelt gratitude to the following people: my mom Ruby Jane, you have made me everything I am today; my dad Nestor-- my eternal, my angel, and the source of my perseverance; Mommyling, my spiritual guide ; Ria & Joe, the true witnesses of my transformation and my foundation pillars; Ellie Jane, the sparkle of our eyes;

Juan, thanks for always encouraging me to push harder - you are my ONE; Rocco & Radha, my reason for everything.

The Love of my family and friends is the fountain of inspiration that never runs dry. Thank you for constantly inspiring me, motivating me, and loving me unconditionally.

This book will never be complete without the help of my trusted and talented friends the #NOWsuperstars and my #oilbularya friends

Blending Essential Oils to use for a very specific reason has become very popular in the recent years. There are several reasons why this is so. Blending EOs is basically about inhaling - as it has been proven that aromas have the ability to trigger feelings, emotions and personal memories.

With this in mind, it is obvious that everyone is unique when it comes to what triggers your senses. It all boils down to personal preference for the aroma to trigger what you want to unleash. Everyone is different and we all connect to the aroma differently, so what might work for one might not work for another person.

Of course, we also want the blend we personalize to be therapeutic. This is the best reason why to blend essential oils. We want the blend we create to help us with a very specific emotion or physical condition. As much as smelling good is important in a blend, it is more important that we blend oils that is not only pleasing to the smell but also produces the therapeutic effect we are after.

Then you have to think about contraindications. Making sure the blend you create is safe to use.

I suggest that before blending find out if the oils you are using is safe for a condition you may have example, if you are pregnant, or have specific allergies. Consult your physician prior to moving forward.

The recipes I have in this book is a compilation of what has proven to work and favored by hundreds of EO enthusiasts. It takes out the guesswork to get you started.

Again, we urge you to read the recipes and make sure that this is safe for you to try.

The book is very specific to a physical and emotional condition. There are several recipes here because you might want to rotate and you may like one and not the other. There is also a variety of application. Some of us prefer to diffuse, some to make roller bottles, and others to create sprays.

I hope you enjoy this compilation, feel free to use the notes section and jot down your fave blends. There is a wonderful world of EO blending - this is just the beginning.

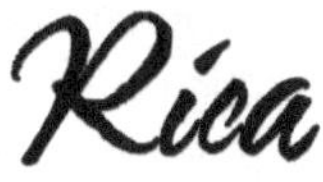

Coughs and Colds are usually caused by a number of things like seasonal allergies, weather change, and/ or viruses. Contributing factors for causing a cough could also be the flu or a common cold. Coughs are not only physically annoying but coughing causes irritation in your lungs, which usually causes more coughing, which could elevate a common cold into an infection.

Persistent coughing could be caused by a number of things like a long-term respiratory tract infection, like chronic bronchitis. Post Nasal Drip – caused by mucus trickling down your throat from the back of the nose, usually stemming from rhinitis or sinusitis.

Usually EOs don't cure the cough, what it does is assist in taming the symptoms that are connected to the cough, the common cold and seasonal allergies. Essential Oils help relieve symptoms of a cough or cold by soothing the throat, combating bacteria, and controlling inflammation.

It could aid to clear your lungs and help fast-track the healing process, making them amazing for dealing with the symptoms.

Why use Essential oils for cough & cold and how can it help?

Viruses are seasonal and at any point in the year it becomes rampant and could cause cough and cold. EOs help in combatting these illnesses and fight allergies. it also strengthens your immune system. In the event you have already been stricken, they can assist in healing faster. The versatility of EOs allows us to use it in many different ways and apply in a variety of ways, giving us multiple options for intervention that best help in healing symptoms or the illness itself.

Since most cough & cold and other respiratory issues are usually caused by viruses, Essential oils' antiviral properties can be great in actually preventing a cough before it even starts to happen.

Table of Contents

Due to climate change, there are also changes in the weather patterns. These changes cause bad health conditions due to the adaptability of our body. To be specific, it primarily affects our respiratory system especially if our immune system is not boosted. Common examples of the sickness we get from climate changes are cough, cold, flu, and others. Let us all admit that cough and cold are pretty much irritating and give us discomfort anywhere we are. These ailments also disrupt us from our slumber for some instance. Everyone has different ways of medication, may it be through prescribed medicines or herbal medicines. However, with the modern medicine, researchers utilized the technology to develop natural treatment, the rise of essential oils. There are a plethora of essential oils in the market, but since we aim to help individuals who suffer from respiratory ailments, we listed some of the most recommended essential oils for cough and cold.

Eucalyptus

We can't deny the fact that eucalyptus oil is recognized for its ability to treat respiratory ailments such as cough. It helps you clean the microorganisms and toxins in your body as it acts as an expectorant. It also helps you fight the bacteria that cause your cough and cold since it has a antimicrobial effect. Eucalyptus may also help relieve muscle pain and tension, and inflammation resulting from cold, cough, or flu.

For inhalation process, add 10-15 drops of eucalyptus essential oil to a bowl of boiling water. Just simply breathe in the vaporized soothing scent for at least 5-10 minutes while it tries to calm and clear you nasal cavity. You may also try to mix a drop of eucalyptus oil and 3 drops of lavender oil in cup of hot water, dampen a washcloth in the mixture and directly apply to your forehead as the lavender oil can also calm your body and mind. One common product of the eucalyptus essential oil is Vicks Vapor Rub, which you can buy in drugstores and pharmacies.

Peppermint

Because of peppermint's antibacterial and antiviral properties, it is considered as one of the top essential oils for cough and cold. This herb contains menthol. Menthol is best known for the relief it gives for congestion so it improves your nasal airflow by unclogging your sinuses. It also gives a cooling sensation which soothes your scratchy throat. Most importantly, it reduces the severity of your cough which gives discomfort.

You may enjoy these peppermint oil benefits in several ways. Have 3-5 drops of peppermint essential oil in a diffuser as it disperses the vaporized soothing scent as it clears your air passage. You can also topically apply 2-3 drops of the oil to the back of your neck and temples, and chest. If you want to create your own vapor rub, try to mix this oil with eucalyptus essential oil for a more satisfying experience. An important note to observe, do not apply near your eyes as it causes irritation.

Rosemary
Rosemary contains cineole, the same substance you can find in eucalyptus which reduces the severity and frequency of cough. The compound cineole also help in breaking the mucus and is a remedy for inflammation. This essential oil boosts the immune system because of its antimicrobial and antioxidant properties. Rosemary also relaxes the muscles in the trachea giving you a respiratory relief.
For topical application, have 5 drops of rosemary essential oil and directly apply to your chest. Inhalation process is pretty common too so you can just simply inhale a diluted rosemary oil for a faster relief. For best results, try combining this oil with either peppermint or eucalyptus essential oil. In a recent research, mixture of these oils helped patients with their cold, cough, and sore throat through inhalation process. Just do it 5 times a day for a few minutes and wait for the favorable results after at least 3 days.

Tea Tree

When essential oils were not yet developed, crushed leaves from tea tree oil were used in treating cough, cold, and congestion. Tea tree has many uses and luckily it can also be used as an essential oil for cough and cold. It is best recognized due to its antibacterial, antiseptic, and antimicrobial properties. It has a vitalizing scent and best works in alleviating congestion resulting from cold. It is a powerful protectant against bacteria, which prevents you from having cold and other respiratory symptoms.

Tea tree essential oil as multipurpose oil comes in many way to be enjoyed. First, you can have a few drops in a diffuser to alleviate chest congestion. You may also have a generous amount to be directly applied to the back of your neck and temple to relieve headache and chronic cough. You may also add a few drops of tea tree oil to a bowl of warm water, soak a towel in the mixture and drape across your chest or head.

Oregano

Oregano contains a compound called carvacrol. In preliminary research, carvacrol was revealed to have interesting results against cancer cells. It expedited cancer cell death, and at the same time remained nontoxic. But on the later studies, health-promoting benefits of carvacrol when it comes to respiratory symptoms were also proven. Carvacrol can fight off various types of germs as it acts as an antimicrobial agent. It also exhibits antiviral activity, which is very much beneficial in relieving respiratory conditions which may lead to cold and cough.

To enjoy the benefits of oregano essential oil through topical application, rub 2-3 drops of the oil mixed with a carrier oil like coconut oil and directly apply to your chest, back, or bottoms of your feet. If you feel symptoms or bacterial conditions which may lead to cough, add a drop or two to a glass of warm water and drink twice daily. However, it was suggested that internal usage of oregano essential oil must be maximized for two week.

The quest for developing natural treatment for different illnesses and ailments never stopped. And since change is constant, our adaptability to external conditions must be stronger. I am referring to our body's adaptability to changes in the weather conditions, to somehow avoid sickness. But as everyone would say, cough and cold is inevitable and might really attack you sometime of the year. If you catch one, try these essential oils for cough and cold mentioned above. They are easy to use and cause minimal side effects. And since prevention is better than cure, just take your daily vitamins.

It is also worth mentioning that the following oils are worth checking out for cough and cold : **Lemon, Lavender, Lemongrass, Peppermint , Cinnamon, Clove, Basil, Juniper, Thyme, Clary Sage, Ginger and Rosemary**

The Blending Process

These EOs are categorized by aromas, and EOs from the same group usually blend fantastically together.

- Floral – Lavender, Geranium, Jasmine
- Woodsy – Pine, Cedarwood
- Earthy – Vetiver, Patchouli
- Herbaceous – Marjoram, Rosemary, Basil
- Minty – Peppermint, Spearmint, Wintergreen
- Medicinal – Eucalyptus, Frankincense, Melaleuca
- Spicy – Pepper, Clove, Cinnamon
- Oriental – Ginger, Patchouli
- Citrus – Wild Orange, Lemon, Lime

Select oils that will give you with the health benefits you are looking to remedy. For increased energy choose: Grapefruit, Lemon, Orange, or Citrus. For Calming and Relaxation choose: Lavender, Cedarwood, or Chamomile. You are encouraged to experiment and play with your oils to see which blends work for you.

TIPS:

- Combine Floral EOs with Woodsy, Spicy and Citrus aromas
- Minty EOs with Woodsy, Earthy, Herbaceous and Citrus aromas
- Earthy EOs with Woodsy and Minty aromas
- Citrus EOs with Floral, Woodsy, Minty, Spicy and Oriental aromas

Diffuse

Diffusing Essential Oils is the safest method to enjoy Essential Oils without the risk of an allergic reaction.

Diffusing Essential Oils
Some Tidbits You Need To Know

Our sense of smell is one of our most powerful senses, and as you have noticed in your own experience that some scents affect your more positively in your minds than others. The body contains over 1,000 receptors for smell—way more receptors than for any of our other senses.

Diffusion Essential Oils means the process vaporizes oils into air by releasing tiny amounts into the air. Inhalation is totally safe and is super low risk. Chances of any EO rising to dangerous levels while diffusion is slim to none.

Diffusing Essential Oils around newborns, babies, young children, pregnant or nursing women, and pets should be done with caution. Read up on safety.

It is advisable that Diffusing Essential Oils for only about 15-30 minutes at a time to be most effective. NEVER leave your diffuser on overnight. Make sure your diffuser is filled with the right amount of water and you understand the operating directions.

While diffusing essential oils, be sure that your space has great ventilation. Crack a window open if the scent become to strong.

Never add Carrier Oils to your diffuser. This may cause your diffuser to malfunction. Clean your diffuser at least 3 times a week with warm water and natural soap to ensure the diffuser is well maintained and bacteria and mold does not accumulate.

Diffusing Essential Oils
Basic Guidelines

Just a few things you need to know and prepare before getting started Diffusing Essential Oils.

Things you need:
Ultrasonic Oil Diffuser
Essential Oils
Water

Just follow the number of drops in the recipe, drop on to an oil diffuser and fill the rest with water.

All diffusers are different and will have its own water minimum and maximum level. Read the diffuser instruction before use.

Ideally, it is best to diffuse for 15-30 minutes and turn off the diffuser. The effect should be good for at least 2-3 hours. Turn your diffuser back on after 3 hours to reinforce oil diffusing effects.

It is not advisable to use EO in humidifiers.

These are not made to release EOS

Diffuser Recipes

Here's a thought for you:

You may be wondering how aroma can simply eliminate symptoms. There's a simple answer to this : Aroma is simply a by-product of diffusing. It's the added benefit but in reality the real benefit comes from the air we breathe and how the body easily absorbs the essential oils released in the air. It works 2 ways, not only does it improve the air quality you breath by disinfecting and eliminating pollutants it also allows your glands to absorb the healing elements of the EOs released in the air molecules,

So for here are a few recipes that can help you manage symptoms and actual issues regarding the matter :

3 Drops Lemon
3 Drops Scotch Pine
3 Drops Lavender
1 Drop Peppermint

----

3 Drops Juniper Berry
4 Drops Rosemary
4 Drops Frankincense

----

4 Drops Cypress
6 Drops Grapefruit

----

5 Drops Cedarwood
4 Drops Lavender
1 Drop Chamomile
1 Drop Eucalyptus (optional)

5-7 Drops Pine or Cedarwood
5-7 Drops Lavender
4 Drops Eucalyptus
1 Drop Lemon

3-5 Drops Rosemary
2 Drops Thyme
1 Drop Peppermint

----

3 Drops Peppermint
3 Drops Lemon
3 Drops Eucalyptus

----

2 Drops Oregano
2 Drops Tea Tree
2 Drops Peppermint
2 Drops Lavender
2 Drops Lemon

3 Drops Tea Tree
2 Drops Lavender
2 Drops Peppermint

----

4 Drops Lavender
4 Drops Peppermint
2 Drops Frankincense
2 Drops Basil

----

3 Drops Rosemary
2 Drops Eucalyptus
2 Drops Peppermint
1 Drops Cypress
1 Drops Lemon

----

2 Drops Lemon
1 Drops Lime
2 Drops Peppermint
1 Drops Rosemary
2 Drops Eucalyptus
1 Drop Clove

----

3 Drops RC
3 Drops Lemon
3 Drops Purification

----

2 Drops Eucalyptus
1 Drops Peppermint

3 Drops Frankincense

----

4 Drops Thieves
3 Drops Eucalyptus Radiata
3 Drops Lavender

----

1 Drop Lemon
1 Drop Eucalyptus
2 Drops Peppermint
1 Drop Rosemary

----

1 Drop Rosemary
2 Drops Eucalyptus
2 Drops Lime
1 Drop Peppermint
1 Drops Frankincense

----

2 Drops Frankincense
2 Drops Orange
1 Drop Eucalyptus

2 Drops Oregano
2 Drops Rosemary
2 Drops Peppermint
2 Drops Eucalyptus

----

3 Drops Eucalyptus
2 Drops Lavender
2 Drop Peppermint

----

3 Drops Eucalyptus
3 Drops Tea Tree

----

4 Drops Eucalyptus
2 Drops Myrrh
4 Drops Cedarwood

----

4 Drops Eucalyptus
2 Drops Ginger
4 Drops Rosemary

----

4 Drops Tea Tree
4 Drops Eucalyptus

Roll

Essential Oil Roller Bottles is the easiest method to enjoy Essential Oils Anywhere and Whenever.

Blending Essential Oils in a Roller Bottle
Some Tidbits You Need To Know

Essential Oils are usually super concentrated and too hard to measure how much to actually put straight from the bottle.

Roller bottles are a way that you are able to create blends ready to use with the right dilution. It allows your EO to last longer.

It also makes it easier to apply exactly where you want to target without getting it all over the place.

It is handy and easy to carry in your purse, ready to use at any time you want to.

I like to apply EOs at the bottom of the feet for many reasons. Our feet have bigger pores than any other skin in our bodies. this means that they are able to suck in the therapeutic compounds in our blend into the bloodstream faster that any other parts of the body. Imagine comparing a normal straw to an oversized straw and how much more you can suck in with the latter. This is how the soles of our feet is compared to the rest of the skin in our bodies.

The skin on our feet is also less sensitive and is designed to withstand some abuse. The risk of having an irritation from EOS is less likely to happen when applied on the feet.

The feet don't have the glands that act as a barrier. Sebaceous glands are glands in our skin that produces an oily substance called Sebum, for the purpose of lubricating and waterproofing the skin. Since this is oil and if you put oil on top of oil, it can act as a barrier or it may slow down penetration.

The feet and palms of our hands are the only skin that don't have these, so it is ideal to apply Essential Oils to the feet for maximum penetration.

Now, it would be hard to apply oils directly and very mess, right? Roller bottles make it super easy and convenient to roll the EOs at the bottom of our feet.

Carrier Oils Info

Carrier oils are vegetable-based oils with their own healing properties that dilute essential oils used to help carry the EOs into the skin.

Essential oils are highly concentrated and could evaporate very quickly. The carrier oil is mixed with the essential oil so it could penetrate the skin before it actually evaporates. Although EOs are oils, it is actually not that oily. When mixed with a carrier oil, it allows you to have more of the essential oil into your skin without wasting EOS to evaporate, making the healing properties of the EO strong and more effective.

There are also Essential oils that are too strong to apply directly to the skin and may cause damage, so it is important to dilute them with a carrier oil.

Never add Carrier Oils to your diffuser. This may cause your diffuser to malfunction. Clean your diffuser at least 3 times a week with warm water and natural soap to ensure the diffuser is well maintained and bacteria and mold does not accumulate.

Carrier Oils

There are a lot of different carrier oils that you can use with EOs to dilute them in a roller bottle.

To name a few :

Almond Oil - moisturizing and stays liquid at room temperature. Do not use if you are allergic to nuts.

Apricot Kernel Oil - moisturizing and suitable for sensitive skin or kids. It is super gentle on the skin.

Avocado Oil - moisturizing and suitable for sensitive and damaged skin. Perfect for skin problems.Can be mixed with other carrier oils

Castor Oil - with antibacterial, antiviral and antifungal properties, use topically to eliminate pain and relieve skin irritation.

Coconut Oil - its antibacterial, antiviral and antifungal properties it is the best and most versatile for skin care. The skin absorbs this very quickly. It solidifies in room temp and may still have a slight coconut oil aroma in it - but you can get a fractionated coconut oil to eliminate the 2 challenges above.

Grapeseed Oil - not just for cooking but also great for topical application on the skin.

Jojoba Oil - one of my faves for skin care blends. This oil is the closest to our natural oil our skin produces to it is absorbed easily without being oily. Also amazing for massage oil blends.

Olive Oil - this is the oil for herb type oils. mostly used for cooking but can also be applied to the skin but would need to be blended with a carrier oil that is mild and absorb well with the skin.

Rosehip Seed Oil - super good for deep moisturizing or skin irritations. This oil has a high content of antioxidants and helps remedy dry, scarred and wounded skin.

Recommended Roller Bottle Dilution Guide

RECOMMENDED ROLL-ON BOTTLE DILUTION AMOUNTS

5 ml (1/6 oz.) Roll-on Bottle = ~100 drops (1tsp.)
10 ml (1/3 oz.) Roll-on Bottle = ~200 drops (2 tsp.)
30 ml. (1 oz.) Roll-on Bottle = ~600 drops (6 tsp.)

Roll-on Size	5 ml	10 ml	30 ml	Add EO drops to roll-on, then fill with carrier oil.	Dilution Percentage
Essential Oil Drops	1	2	6	1%	
	2	4	12	2%	
	3	6	18	3%	
	5	10	30	5%	
	10	20	60	10%	
	20	40	120	20%	
	25	50	150	25%	
	50	100	300	50%	

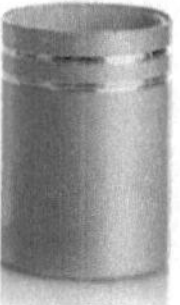

General Guidelines:
Birth to 12 months = .3-.5% dilution
1-5 years = 1.5-3% dilution
6-11 years = 1.5-5% dilution
12-17 years = 1.5-20% dilution
18 years and older = 1.5% dilution-Neat (no dilution)
Elderly or Sensitive Skin = 1-3% dilution
Daily Use = 2-5% dilution
Short Term Use = 10-25% dilution
Local Skin or Systemic Issues = 50% dilution-Neat

These are general guidelines suggestions--not absolute rules--based on traditional aromatheraphy practice.
(Kurt Schnaubelt PhD, Valerie Worwood, Robert Tisserand)

Dilution Basics:

How much you dilute your EO depends on different factors such as weight, sensitivity, health conditions, EOs that are blended in or how long that blend has been used for. There is never an absolute dilution rule, it is you who knows about your level and tolerance. I feel that it is best to start with a higher dilution percentage and increase EO drops over time.

To make sure your EO is safe, make sure that the oils you use are therapeutic grade and do your research on the source and extraction methods used to produce the oils.

Roller Bottle Blending Order

I normally just start with dropping the drops of oils into the **10mL roller bottle**, then adding the carrier oil up until the shoulder of the bottle. Capping the bottle off with the roller and the bottle cap. Instead of shaking the bottle, i like to roll the bottle between my palms first for a minute or 2 for blending, then finishing it off with a few shakes.

NOTE: All recipes in this book is for a 10mL Roller Bottle. If you have a bigger or smaller roller bottle, adjust the number of EO drops based on the size of your bottle.

Roller Bottle Recipes

4 drops Onguard
4 drops Oregano
4 drops Lemon

----

10 drops Respiratory Blend
6 drops Lime

----

5 drops Eucalyptus
3 drops Frankincense
2 drops Lemon

----

8 drops Breathe
5 drops Lime

----

6 drops Respiratory Blend
4 drops Eucalyptus
3 drops Frankincense

----

4 drops Lemon
4 drops Peppermint
2 drops Frankincense

----

6 drops RC
4 drops Lemon
4 drops Purification
2 drops Thyme

----

3 drops Lemon
3 drops Clove
3 drops Eucalyptus
3 drops Rosemary

----

4 drops Oregano
6 drops Lemon
5 drops On Guard
5 drops Melaleuca

----

4 drops Frankincense
4 drops Lemon
4 drops Melaleuca Tea Tree
4 drops Protective Blend

----

2 drops Oregano
2 drops Melaleuca
2 drops Lemon
2 drops Frankincense
2 drops Cinnamon

----

3 drops Orange
3 drops Lemon
3 drops Thieves
3 drops Frankincense

----

4 drops Thieves

4 drops Purification
4 drops Oregano

----

8 drops Respiratory Blend
5 drops Eucalyptus
4 drops Frankincense

----

6 drop Cardamom
6 drop Frankincense

----

2 drops Oregano
2 drops Tea Tree
2 drops Lemon
2 drops Frankincense
2 drops Cinnamon

----

4 drops Peppermint
2 drops Eucalyptus
2 drops Lemon
2 drops Rosemary

----

2 drops Lemon
6 drops Lavender
2 drops Peppermint

----

4 drops Peace & Calming
3 drops Lavender

3 drops Frankincense

Bonus Recipes

Pain Relief Massage Oil Favorite

60mL Jojoba Oil (cold pressed)
8 drops Lavender
8 drops Peppermint
15 drops Frankincense

Pain Relief Massage Oil Secret

14 drops Frankincense
10 drops Sweet Orange
8 drops Turmeric
30mL Sweet Almond Oil

Pain Relief Bath Soak Blend

10 drops Frankincense
5 drops Lavender
5 drops Bergamot
1 cup Full-Cream/ Full-Fat Milk

Pain Relief Bath Salt Blend

1 cup Epsom Salt
¼ cup Dead Sea Salt
¼ cup Baking Soda
8-10 drops Essential Oils
(use any ingredient above or single oils)

Inhale

Essential Oil Inhalers are the most convenient way to enjoy Essential Oils Anywhere and Whenever.

Essential Oil Inhalers give you quick and easy access to the vast therapeutic benefits of essential oils.

Blending Essential Oils in an Inhaler Some Tidbits You Need To Know

EO Inhalers or aroma sticks are compact tubes, with a cotton wick inside and a protective cover, to lock the aroma within.

Your preferred blend of essential oils is absorbed by the cotton wick, and safely enclosed in a tube that that fits inside of the cover. The cover is easily removed for access to the tube to breathe in the aroma. Usually lasts about 3 months, depending on the oil blend used.

I absolutely love these because they encourage me to take a moment during super stressful moments, and just breathe.

It is in times of stress when our breathing patterns often change and taking deep breaths promote a feeling of calm and inner peace. Breath work combined with visualization plus a relaxing inhaler, can offer relief to symptoms of stress and help your body to come back to the state of homeostasis.

Aroma Sticks can be carried in your tiny purse, even compact enough to fit in your pocket. You can enjoy your favorite EOs anywhere and you can use them with discretion.

I love diffusing, and do all the time but not everyone in my space may enjoy the scents I enjoy or they may not benefit from the therapeutic benefits of the EOs I am diffusing - so the inhaler is one way to not only enjoy my choice of blends but to keep in personal not affecting everyone else around me.

Inhalers not only benefits me but also keep those around me safe in case the oils I want to blend may pose a risk to those around me who may have health issue not advised to be exposed to my choice EOs/

When making Aroma Sticks, You may use your chosen EOs at 100% Concentration.

Inhaler Basic Guidelines

Breathe in slow and deep to absorb the EO molecules directly into your olfactory system.

Inhalers are super easy to use. You just remove the cap and inhale from the inhaler tube, count 1 to 5 slowly as you inhale. The EO molecules get drawn into our bloodstream through our nasal cavity and gets delivered throughout our entire body.

Simple to use, easy to cary, portable and compact. You never have to be without your favorite blends, ever.

Inhaler Blending Basics

Inhalers are super easy and simple to make.

All you need is an inhaler set which consist of the following:

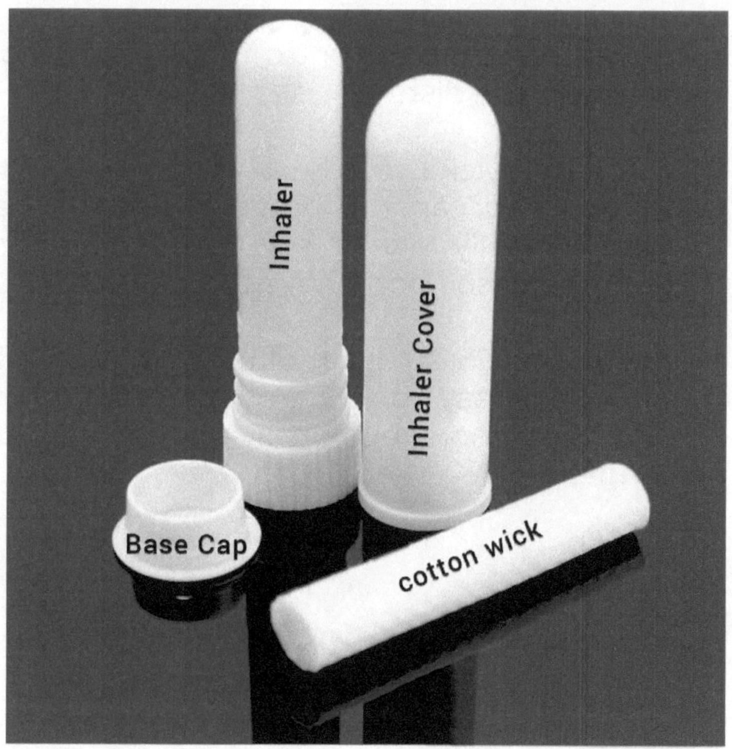

Inhaler, Inhaler Cover, Base Cap and Cotton Wick.

You will need your Essential Oils.

I like to use a pipette for precision and a small petri dish so I can see the oil.

Blending is super easy, just combine the drops and swirl it around in the petri dish and when you are satisfied you can go ahead and drop the cotton wick to absorb all the oil in the dish.

Once the wick is ready you can drop it in the inhaler and cap the bottom with the Base Cap. I usually like to secure the cover with the inhaler so I don't have to do it later.

I usually us 15-20 drops of EO total in a recipe and it can last up to 3 months. Some recipes will need more but on average it is in this range.

Inhaler Recipes

6 drops of Balance
4 drops of Eucalyptus
3 drops of Lemon
2 drops of Lime

----

5 drops of Frankincense
6 drops of Lavender
4 drops of Wild Orange

----

5 drops RC
2 drops Peppermint
2 drops Frankincense

----

3 drops of Lavender
3 drops of Lemon
3 drops of Melrose
3 drops of Eucalyptus
3 drops of RC
3 drops of Peppermint
3 drops of Copaiba

----

2 drop of Lemon
4 drops of Eucalyptus Radiata
6 drops of Rosemary
4 drops of Peppermint

----

4 drops of Peppermint
4 drops of Eucalyptus
2 drops of Lavender
2 drops of Lemon
2 drops of Rosemary

----

4 drops of Eucalyptus
4 drops of Siberian Fir
4 drops of Peppermint

----

9 drops Rosemary
3 drop Thyme
3 drop Peppermint

5-7 drops of Pine or Cedarwood
5-7 drops of Lavender
4 drops of Eucalyptus
1 drop of Lemon

----

8 drops of Rosemary
8 drops of Peppermint
6 drops of Eucalyptus

----

10 drops of Rosemary
4 drops of Thyme
2 drop of Peppermint

----

6 drops of Pine or Rosemary
6 drops of Peppermint
4 drops of Eucalyptus

----

9 drops of Rosemary
3 drop of Thyme
3 drop of Peppermint

----

3 drops of Oregano
3 drops of Tea Tree
3 drops of Lemon
3 drops of Frankincense
3 drops of Cinnamon Leaf

----

6 drops of Spruce
4 drops of Eucalyptus
3 drops of Lemon
2 drops of Lime

----

5 drops of Frankincense
6 drops of Lavender
4 drops of Wild Orange

----

6 drops of Eucalyptus
3 drops of Roman Chamomile
6 drops of Frankincense

----

4 drops of Cedarwood
6 drops of Roman Chamomile
10 drops of Frankincense

----

8 drops of Thieves
4 drops of Frankincense
4 drops of Lemon

----

5 drops of Lemon
5 drops of Lavender
5 drops of Peppermint

----

3 drops of Oregano
3 drops of Tea Tree
3 drops of Lemon
3 drops of Frankincense
3 drops of Cinnamon

----

9 drops of Hyssop
5 drops of Black Spruce
3 drops of Lavender
1 drop of Peppermint

----

3 drop of Black Spruce
6 drops of Lavender
6 drops of Scotch Pine
3 drop of Spearmint

<u>Book Ordering</u>

To order your copy / copies of
Essential Oils
for Cough and Cold

please visit: **EOrecipes.net**

You can also check out other titles available.

Bulk Pricing and
Affiliate Programs Available